FUNCTIONAL FITNESS

For Seniors

A Comprehensive Guide To Strength, Mobility, And Balance Exercises For Healthy Aging, Increased Energy, And Improved Quality Of Life

ROBERT LUGO

Introduction	4
CHAPTER 1	**12**
Understanding Functional Fitness	12
CHAPTER 2	**19**
Functional Movement Patterns	19
CHAPTER 3	**23**
Core Stability And Strength	23
CHAPTER 4	**32**
Mobility And Flexibility Training	32
CHAPTER 5	**36**
Integrating Cardiovascular Training	36
CHAPTER 6	**41**
Functional Fitness Equipment	41
CHAPTER 7	**48**
Programming And Periodization	48
CHAPTER 8	**56**
Nutrition For Functional Fitness	56
CHAPTER 9	**60**
Injury Prevention And Recovery	60
CHAPTER 10	**67**
Monitoring Progress And Goal Setting	67
CHAPTER 11	**74**
Advanced Functional Training Techniques	74

CHAPTER 12 81
   Mental Conditioning And Mindfulness 81

CHAPTER 13 88
   Special Populations And Functional Fitness.....................88
   Conclusion 91

Introduction

What is Functional Fitness?

Functional fitness is a dynamic approach to exercise that focuses on training the body to perform daily tasks and activities with efficiency and ease. Unlike traditional workout routines that often isolate muscle groups or focus solely on aesthetics, functional fitness emphasizes movements that mimic real-life activities such as bending, lifting, pushing, pulling, and rotating. The goal is to improve overall physical functionality, mobility, stability, and strength in ways that translate directly to improved performance in everyday life.

At the core of functional fitness is the concept of functional movement patterns, which involve multi-joint, multi-muscle exercises that holistically engage the body. These movements enhance coordination, balance, flexibility, and endurance while promoting joint health and reducing the risk of injuries. Functional fitness workouts are often dynamic, varied, and adaptable, making them suitable for individuals of all fitness levels and ages.

Benefits of Functional Fitness:

The benefits of functional fitness extend beyond the gym walls, influencing various aspects of daily life and overall well-being. Some key benefits include:

1.   Improved Functional Capacity: Functional fitness enhances your ability to perform everyday tasks more efficiently and with less effort. Whether it's carrying groceries, lifting objects, or playing with children, increased functional capacity makes daily activities feel easier and less strenuous.

2.   Enhanced Core Strength and Stability: Many functional exercises engage the core muscles, including the abdominals, obliques, and lower back. A strong and stable core is essential for maintaining proper posture, preventing back

pain, and supporting overall body alignment and movement.

3. Increased Joint Mobility and Flexibility: Functional movements involve a wide range of motion in multiple joints, promoting joint mobility, flexibility, and range of motion. This can improve joint health, reduce stiffness, and enhance overall movement quality.

4. Functional Muscle Development: Functional fitness workouts target multiple muscle groups simultaneously, promoting balanced muscle development and functional strength. This contrasts with isolated exercises that focus on specific muscles but may neglect overall functional capacity.

5. Injury Prevention: By training the body in functional movement patterns, functional fitness helps improve movement mechanics, reduce imbalances, and strengthen stabilizing muscles. This can lower the risk of injuries during daily activities and sports participation.

6. Adaptability and Variety: Functional fitness workouts are highly adaptable and can be tailored to individual needs, goals, and fitness levels. They offer a variety of exercises, equipment options, and workout formats, keeping workouts engaging, challenging, and effective.

7. Improved Quality of Life: The practical benefits of functional fitness, such as increased energy, mobility, and independence, contribute to an improved quality of life. Whether it's navigating stairs with ease, participating in recreational activities, or maintaining an active lifestyle as you age, functional fitness supports overall well-being.

Importance of Functional Movement Patterns:

Functional movement patterns form the foundation of functional fitness, defining how the body moves efficiently and effectively in real-world scenarios. These patterns involve coordination between multiple joints, muscles, and body segments to perform tasks such as squatting, lunging, pushing, pulling, twisting, and carrying.

Understanding and incorporating functional movement patterns into your workout routine offers several advantages:

1. Natural Movement Replication: Functional movement patterns mimic the natural movements we perform daily, making them highly relevant and practical for improving real-life functionality.

2. Whole-Body Integration: Functional movements engage multiple muscle groups and joints simultaneously, promoting holistic movement patterns and overall body integration. This leads to improved coordination, balance, and movement efficiency.

3. Transferability to Daily Activities: By training in functional movement patterns, you develop skills and strength that directly transfer to everyday activities like lifting objects, bending, reaching, and maintaining stability during various tasks.

4.   Core Activation and Stability: Many functional movements require core activation and stability, strengthening the muscles that support the spine, pelvis, and torso. This not only improves posture but also reduces the risk of back pain and injuries.

5.   Joint Health and Flexibility: Functional movement patterns promote joint mobility, flexibility, and range of motion, which are essential for joint health, injury prevention, and optimal movement mechanics.

6.   Functional Strength Development: Functional movements emphasize functional strength, which is the ability to generate force and control movements in real-world situations. This type of strength is practical and applicable to daily tasks and activities.

Target Audience for this Manual:

The target audience for this manual on functional fitness includes individuals of all ages and fitness levels who are interested in improving their overall physical functionality, movement quality, and well-being. This includes:

1. Beginners to Fitness: Those who are new to exercise or fitness training and want to start with a functional approach that enhances daily functionality and movement patterns.

2. Fitness Enthusiasts: Individuals who are already active or have experience in fitness training and want to explore the benefits of functional fitness for improved performance and injury prevention.

3. Active Aging Population: Older adults who seek to maintain independence, mobility, and quality of life by incorporating functional exercises that support daily activities and functional capacity.

4. Athletes and Sports Enthusiasts: Athletes and sports enthusiasts looking to enhance their athletic performance, movement efficiency, and injury resilience through functional training principles.

5. Rehabilitation and Injury Prevention: Individuals recovering from injuries or seeking to prevent injuries by improving movement mechanics, joint stability, and functional strength.

6. Health and Wellness Seekers: Those interested in holistic health and wellness, including mental, emotional, and physical well-being, through functional fitness practices that promote overall functional capacity and vitality.

This manual provides comprehensive guidance, exercises, and strategies for incorporating functional fitness into daily routines, regardless of the individual's starting point or fitness background. It aims to empower readers to optimize their movement patterns, functional strength, and overall health through practical, evidence-based approaches to fitness training.

CHAPTER 1
Understanding Functional Fitness

Functional fitness is a dynamic and multifaceted approach to exercise that aims to enhance one's ability to perform daily activities and meet the demands of everyday life effectively.

At its core, functional fitness emphasizes movements that mimic real-life activities, focusing on improving strength, flexibility, coordination, balance, and endurance holistically.

This section delves into the key concepts of understanding functional fitness, including its definition, principles, and historical evolution.

Definition of Functional Fitness

Functional fitness is defined as a form of training that emphasizes exercises and movements that directly contribute to improving one's ability to perform activities of daily living (ADLs) with ease and efficiency.

Unlike traditional gym workouts that often isolate specific muscle groups or focus solely on aesthetics, functional fitness programs target functional movement patterns that are relevant to everyday tasks such as bending, lifting, pushing, pulling, and twisting.

The cornerstone of functional fitness is its practicality and applicability to real-life scenarios. Rather than aiming for a particular body shape or size, the goal is to develop functional strength, mobility, and endurance that translate into improved performance in various activities, whether at home, work, or during recreational pursuits.

Principles of Functional Fitness

1. Functional Movement Patterns: Functional fitness exercises are designed to mimic natural movement patterns that the body regularly performs. These movements typically involve multiple joints and muscle groups working together in a coordinated manner.

2. Multi-Planar Movement: Functional fitness training incorporates movements in multiple planes of motion (sagittal, frontal, and transverse planes) to enhance overall mobility and stability. This multidimensional approach ensures that the body is prepared for a wide range of movements in daily life.

3. Core Stability and Strength: A strong and stable core is essential for functional fitness.

Core exercises target the muscles of the abdomen, lower back, and pelvis, providing a solid foundation for performing everyday activities and maintaining proper posture.

4. Balance and Coordination: Functional fitness programs include exercises that improve balance and coordination, reducing the risk of falls and enhancing agility and motor skills.

These exercises often integrate proprioceptive and neuromuscular training techniques.

5. Progressive Overload: Like any effective fitness regimen, functional fitness employs the

principle of progressive overload to stimulate continuous improvements.

This involves gradually increasing the intensity, duration, or complexity of exercises over time to challenge the body and promote adaptation.

6 Individualized Approach: Functional fitness programs can be tailored to individual needs, taking into account factors such as age, fitness level, injury history, and specific goals.

Personalized programming ensures that exercises are safe, effective, and relevant to the individual's lifestyle.

History and Evolution of Functional Fitness

The roots of functional fitness can be traced back to various disciplines and training methodologies that prioritize functional movement and performance.

While the term "functional fitness" gained popularity in recent decades, its principles have long been integrated into diverse fitness modalities and sports training programs.

One of the early influences on functional fitness was the field of physical therapy, which focused on restoring functional abilities and movement patterns in individuals recovering from injuries or surgeries.

Physical therapists recognized the importance of functional exercises that mimic real-world tasks to facilitate rehabilitation and improve overall functional capacity.

In the realm of sports performance, functional training became prominent as athletes and coaches sought ways to enhance athletic performance beyond traditional strength and conditioning methods.

Functional exercises that replicated sport-specific movements and demands were integrated into training protocols to improve agility, speed, power, and injury prevention.

The emergence of functional fitness as a distinct fitness approach gained momentum in the late 20th century and early 21st century, fueled by growing awareness of the limitations of isolated muscle training and the benefits of functional movement patterns.

Fitness professionals, rehabilitation specialists, and exercise enthusiasts embraced the concept of functional fitness as a more holistic and practical approach to fitness and wellness.

Over time, functional fitness evolved to encompass a wide range of modalities and training tools, from bodyweight exercises and functional movement drills to specialized equipment such as stability balls, resistance bands, kettlebells, and suspension trainers.

The integration of functional training principles into mainstream fitness programs further solidified its place as a valuable and effective fitness paradigm for people of all ages and fitness levels.

Understanding functional fitness involves recognizing its focus on practical, movement-based exercises that improve overall functional capacity, its foundational principles that guide training methodologies, and its historical evolution from diverse influences within the realms of rehabilitation, sports performance, and general fitness.

CHAPTER 2
Functional Movement Patterns

Functional Movement Patterns play a crucial role in Functional Fitness, emphasizing movements that mimic daily activities and improve overall functionality.

These patterns encompass a range of movements that are essential for daily living, athletic performance, and injury prevention. Understanding and incorporating Functional Movement Patterns into fitness routines can lead to improved mobility, strength, and coordination.

Squatting Techniques and Variations are foundational to Functional Fitness. The squat is a compound movement that targets multiple muscle groups, including the quadriceps, hamstrings, glutes, and core. Proper squatting technique involves maintaining a neutral spine, engaging the core, and distributing weight evenly through the feet.

Variations such as goblet squats, front squats, and pistol squats provide options to target different muscle groups and add variety to workouts, promoting muscle balance and functional strength.

Hinging Movements, including exercises like deadlifts and kettlebell swings, focus on hip hinge mechanics and posterior chain activation. Deadlifts are effective for strengthening the hamstrings, glutes, and lower back while improving hip mobility and core stability. Kettlebell swings combine strength and cardio benefits, emphasizing explosive hip extension and proper body mechanics. Incorporating hinging movements into a functional fitness routine enhances overall strength, power, and functional movement patterns.

Pushing Exercises, such as push-ups and overhead presses, target the upper body pushing muscles including the chest, shoulders, and triceps. Push-ups are a bodyweight staple that can be modified for different fitness levels, emphasizing core stability and shoulder health.

Overhead press variations using dumbbells or barbells build shoulder strength and stability, promoting functional upper-body strength for activities like lifting and pushing objects overhead.

Pulling Movements are essential for balanced upper body strength and posture. Exercises like rows and pull-ups target the back muscles including the latissimus dorsi, rhomboids, and traps.

Rows can be performed with various equipment such as dumbbells, barbells, or resistance bands, focusing on scapular retraction and shoulder stability. Pull-ups challenge upper body strength and grip, improving functional pulling strength and muscle engagement.

Rotational and Anti-Rotational Exercises add another dimension to functional fitness by targeting rotational stability and core strength.

Rotational exercises like Russian twists, woodchoppers, and cable twists engage the obliques and improve torso rotation for activities that involve twisting or turning movements.

Anti-rotational exercises such as Pallof presses and plank variations challenge core stability and prevent excessive rotation, enhancing overall functional movement control and injury resilience.

In conclusion, Functional Movement Patterns are fundamental to Functional Fitness, encompassing a range of movements that improve mobility, strength, and coordination for daily activities and athletic performance.

Incorporating squatting techniques and variations, hinging movements like deadlifts and kettlebell swings, pushing exercises such as push-ups and overhead presses, pulling movements like rows and pull-ups, and rotational/anti-rotational exercises enhance overall functional fitness and movement quality.

CHAPTER 3
Core Stability And Strength

Core stability and strength are foundational elements in functional fitness, playing a crucial role in overall movement efficiency, injury prevention, and performance enhancement.

The core, often referred to as the body's powerhouse, encompasses muscles in the abdomen, lower back, hips, and pelvis. Its primary function is to provide stability and support for movements in various planes of motion, making it essential for activities ranging from everyday tasks to athletic endeavors. In this section, we delve into the importance of core stability, core exercises for functional fitness, and the progressions and variations that can be implemented to optimize core strength and stability.

Importance of Stability

Core stability is Core the ability of the core muscles to maintain optimal alignment and support while resisting external forces or producing movement. It forms the foundation for efficient movement patterns and contributes significantly to posture, balance, and functional performance. A strong and stable core not only enhances athletic performance but also reduces the risk of injuries, especially those related to the spine and lower extremities.

In functional fitness, where movements are often multi-planar and dynamic, core stability is paramount. It allows individuals to transfer force effectively between the upper and lower body, generating power and control during exercises such as squats, deadlifts, and overhead presses. Furthermore, a stable core enables better control and coordination in movements that involve rotation, flexion, extension, and lateral bending, enhancing overall movement quality and efficiency.

Several factors contribute to core stability, including muscle strength, endurance, neuromuscular control, and intra-abdominal pressure.

Core stability exercises aim to target these factors comprehensively, leading to improved functional performance and reduced injury risk in both athletic and daily life activities.

Core Exercises for Functional Fitness

Core exercises for functional fitness encompass a wide range of movements that target different aspects of core stability and strength.

These exercises can be categorized based on their primary focus, including anti-rotation, anti-extension, anti-flexion, rotation, and stabilization. Incorporating a variety of core exercises into a training program ensures a well-rounded approach to developing core strength and stability.

1. Anti-Rotation Exercises: These exercises focus on resisting rotational forces, which is

crucial for maintaining stability during activities that involve twisting or turning. Examples include Pallof presses, plank rotations, and cable chops.

2. Anti-Extension Exercises: Targeting the ability to resist excessive arching of the lower back, anti-extension exercises help strengthen the anterior core muscles. Movements like plank variations (e.g., forearm plank, high plank), ab wheel rollouts, and dead bugs are effective for building core stability in this plane.

3. Anti-Flexion Exercises: These exercises emphasize preventing excessive rounding of the spine, and strengthening the posterior core muscles. Exercises such as back extensions, reverse hyperextensions, and bird-dog variations are beneficial for developing core stability in the sagittal plane.

4. Rotation Exercises: Rotation exercises involve twisting movements that challenge the obliques and rotational stability of the core. Russian twists, woodchoppers, and medicine ball

twists are examples of exercises that target rotational strength and control.

5. Stabilization Exercises: Stabilization exercises focus on maintaining a neutral spine and pelvis position while performing dynamic movements or holding static positions.

Planks (including side planks), bird dogs, and dead bugs are fundamental stabilization exercises that engage multiple core muscles simultaneously.

In functional fitness programs, these core exercises can be integrated into circuit training, HIIT workouts, or dedicated core training sessions. The selection of exercises should be based on individual fitness levels, goals, and any specific weaknesses or imbalances that need to be addressed.

Progressions and Variations for Core Work

Progressions and variations play a crucial role in advancing core strength and stability over time. Progressions involve increasing the intensity, complexity, or duration of exercises to continue challenging the core muscles and eliciting adaptations. Variations, on the other hand, introduce new movements or equipment to add diversity to core training and target different muscle groups within the core.

1. Progressive Overload: Gradually increasing the difficulty of core exercises is key to ongoing improvement. This can be achieved by adding resistance (e.g., using weights or resistance bands), increasing time under tension, or performing more challenging variations of familiar exercises.

2. Dynamic Movements: Incorporating dynamic movements into core training adds functional relevance and challenges the core in a dynamic, multi-planar manner. Exercises such as mountain climbers, bicycle crunches, and hanging leg raises require coordination, stability, and muscular endurance.

3. Unilateral Exercises: Unilateral exercises, where one side of the body is emphasized, are effective for addressing asymmetries and enhancing core stability. Single-arm plank variations, single-leg deadlifts, and unilateral farmer's carries are examples of unilateral core exercises.

4. Integration with Compound Movements: Integrating core activation into compound movements such as squats, lunges, and overhead presses enhances overall stability and strength. Exercises like the overhead squat, front squat, and kettlebell swing engage the core while targeting other muscle groups simultaneously.

5. Functional Equipment: Utilizing functional fitness equipment like stability balls, resistance bands, kettlebells, and suspension trainers adds variety and challenges the core in different ways. For instance, performing exercises such as stability ball rollouts, band-resisted rotations, kettlebell windmills, or TRX pikes can enhance core strength and stability.

6. Plyometric Exercises: Incorporating plyometric exercises into core training improves power production and reactive strength. Plyo push-ups, medicine ball slams, and box jumps with a rotational component are examples of plyometric exercises that engage the core dynamically.

7. Balance and Proprioception Training: Including exercises that challenge balance and proprioception (awareness of body position) enhances core stability and neuromuscular control. Exercises like single-leg balance with reaches, stability ball exercises, and BOSU ball exercises improve core stability in unstable environments.

By incorporating progressions and variations strategically into core training programs, individuals can continually challenge their core muscles, prevent plateaus, and improve overall functional fitness. It's important to progress gradually, ensuring proper form and technique to maximize benefits and minimize the risk of injury.

In conclusion, core stability and strength are fundamental aspects of functional fitness, contributing significantly to movement efficiency, injury prevention, and performance enhancement. Understanding the importance of core stability, implementing a variety of core exercises, and utilizing progressions and variations are essential strategies for developing a strong and resilient core. Incorporating these principles into functional fitness programs can lead to improved functional capacity, athletic performance, and overall well-being.

CHAPTER 4
Mobility And Flexibility Training

Understanding Mobility vs. Flexibility

Mobility and flexibility are often used interchangeably in fitness discussions, yet they represent distinct aspects of movement.

Flexibility refers to the ability of muscles and connective tissues to stretch passively, allowing for a greater range of motion.

On the other hand, mobility encompasses the range of motion actively achievable by a joint or series of joints.

In simpler terms, flexibility is about the tissues' ability to stretch, while mobility involves how well joints can move through that range.

This differentiation is crucial in functional fitness because it determines not just how far a limb can stretch but how effectively it can be used in dynamic movements.

The Importance of Joint Mobility

Joint mobility is a cornerstone of functional fitness as it directly impacts how efficiently the body can perform various movements. Proper joint mobility enhances athletic performance, reduces the risk of injuries, and promotes overall functional movement patterns. In functional fitness, where movements often involve multiple joints working together, optimal joint mobility ensures smooth and coordinated actions. It allows for better force transmission, stability, and control, all of which are vital for functional tasks like lifting, carrying, pushing, and pulling.

Dynamic Warm-ups for Functional Workouts

Dynamic warm-ups play a pivotal role in preparing the body for functional workouts. Unlike static stretching, which focuses on holding positions to lengthen muscles, dynamic warm-ups involve active movements that mimic the exercises to follow. These movements gradually increase heart rate, blood flow, and body temperature while priming muscles, tendons, and ligaments for dynamic activities. Dynamic warm-ups not only enhance performance but also reduce the risk of injuries by improving joint lubrication, muscle elasticity, and neuromuscular coordination.

Mobility Drills for Key Joints (Shoulders, Hips, Ankles)

Specific mobility drills targeting key joints like shoulders, hips, and ankles are essential for maintaining optimal functional fitness. For the shoulders, exercises such as arm circles, shoulder dislocations, and thoracic spine rotations help improve mobility and stability, crucial for overhead movements and upper body strength.

Hip mobility drills like hip circles, leg swings, and hip flexor stretches enhance flexibility and range of motion, benefiting movements like squats, lunges, and running. Ankles, often neglected yet vital for balance and agility, can be improved through exercises like ankle circles, calf raises, and dorsiflexion stretches, aiding in movements such as jumping, landing, and lateral shifts.

Understanding the difference between mobility and flexibility, prioritizing joint mobility, incorporating dynamic warm-ups, and utilizing targeted mobility drills for key joints are foundational concepts in functional fitness.

These elements not only optimize performance but also contribute to long-term joint health, injury prevention, and overall functional movement proficiency.

CHAPTER 5
Integrating Cardiovascular Training

Cardiovascular training plays a crucial role in enhancing overall fitness and functional capacity. When integrated strategically into functional fitness programs, it can significantly improve endurance, stamina, and cardiovascular health. This section delves into the importance of cardiovascular training in functional fitness, explores the benefits for overall health, and discusses specific methods such as High-Intensity Interval Training (HIIT) and endurance workouts tailored for functional athletes.

Cardiovascular Health and Functional Fitness

Functional fitness encompasses the ability to perform daily tasks efficiently and without undue fatigue. Central to this concept is cardiovascular health, which directly influences one's capacity for sustained physical activity. In the context of functional fitness, cardiovascular training targets the heart and lungs, improving their efficiency in delivering oxygen to muscles and removing waste products during exercise. This leads to enhanced endurance, allowing individuals to engage in prolonged physical activities without exhaustion.

The benefits of cardiovascular training in functional fitness extend beyond endurance. Regular cardiovascular exercise promotes heart health by reducing the risk of cardiovascular diseases such as heart attack, stroke, and hypertension. It also contributes to weight management, as it helps burn calories and improve metabolic function. Furthermore, cardiovascular training enhances overall well-being by boosting mood, reducing stress, and improving sleep quality, factors that are vital for maintaining a healthy lifestyle conducive to functional fitness.

HIIT (High-Intensity Interval Training) for Functional Conditioning

High-Intensity Interval Training (HIIT) has gained popularity for its effectiveness in improving cardiovascular fitness and metabolic function. In a functional fitness context, HIIT offers unique benefits by incorporating intense bursts of activity followed by periods of rest or low-intensity recovery. This approach mimics the demands of real-life activities that require short bursts of high effort, such as sprinting to catch a bus or lifting heavy objects.

The key principle of HIIT is its ability to elicit a high level of cardiovascular stress in a short amount of time. This leads to adaptations such as increased aerobic capacity, improved anaerobic performance, and enhanced overall endurance. For functional athletes, HIIT can be tailored to mimic the demands of their specific activities, whether it's quick bursts of power in sports like basketball or rapid movements in functional training routines.

Endurance Workouts for Functional Athletes

Endurance is a critical component of functional fitness, especially for athletes engaged in activities that require sustained effort over extended periods. Endurance workouts focus on building cardiovascular stamina and the ability to perform repetitive movements without fatigue.

For functional athletes, endurance training is essential for maintaining peak performance during prolonged training sessions or competitions.

Endurance workouts for functional athletes can take various forms, including long-distance running, cycling, swimming, and circuit training. These activities aim to challenge the cardiovascular system while also improving muscular endurance and mental resilience.

By incorporating endurance workouts into their training regimen, functional athletes can enhance their ability to sustain effort during complex movements, maintain technique under fatigue, and recover more efficiently between bouts of activity.

integrating cardiovascular training into functional fitness programs is essential for promoting overall health, enhancing endurance, and supporting the demands of functional activities. Whether through HIIT for intense conditioning or endurance workouts for sustained performance, cardiovascular training plays a vital role in optimizing functional fitness and improving quality of life.

CHAPTER 6
Functional Fitness Equipment

Functional fitness equipment plays a pivotal role in enhancing physical performance, promoting functional movement patterns, and improving overall fitness levels. This section provides a comprehensive overview of various types of functional fitness equipment, including bodyweight exercises and their variations, dumbbells, kettlebells, barbells, and functional training machines and tools such as TRX and resistance bands.

Overview of Functional Fitness Equipment

Functional fitness equipment encompasses a wide range of tools and apparatus designed to facilitate functional movement patterns that mimic real-life activities. Unlike traditional gym equipment that often isolates specific muscle groups, functional fitness equipment emphasizes integrated movements that engage multiple muscle groups simultaneously.

This approach not only enhances muscular strength but also improves coordination, balance, and stability, making it highly beneficial for daily activities and sports performance.

One of the key characteristics of functional fitness equipment is its versatility. Many pieces of equipment can be adjusted or used in various ways to create different resistance levels or movement challenges, making them suitable for individuals of different fitness levels and goals.

Additionally, functional fitness equipment often incorporates elements of instability, requiring users to engage their core muscles and stabilizers for proper execution, further enhancing functional strength and stability.

Bodyweight Exercises and Their Variations

Bodyweight exercises form the foundation of functional fitness training, as they utilize the individual's body weight as resistance.

These exercises not only improve strength but also promote flexibility, mobility, and body awareness. Some common bodyweight exercises include squats, lunges, push-ups, planks, and burpees, each targeting different muscle groups and movement patterns.

Variations of bodyweight exercises add complexity and challenge to workouts, allowing for progression as fitness levels improve. For example, variations of squats include pistol squats, jump squats, and Bulgarian split squats, each requiring greater strength, balance, and coordination. Similarly, push-up variations like diamond push-ups, plyometric push-ups, and decline push-ups target different areas of the chest, shoulders, and triceps, enhancing overall upper body strength.

Dumbbells, Kettlebells, and Barbells in Functional Training

Dumbbells, kettlebells, and barbells are essential tools in functional training, offering a wide range of exercises to target various muscle groups and movement patterns. Dumbbells, with their handheld design, allow for unilateral movements that improve balance and symmetry between both sides of the body. Exercises such as dumbbell squats, lunges, rows, and presses engage multiple muscle groups while challenging stability and coordination.

Kettlebells, characterized by their off-center weight distribution, are particularly effective for dynamic and ballistic movements. Kettlebell swings, snatches, cleans, and Turkish get-ups not only build strength but also enhance power, endurance, and cardiovascular fitness. The unique shape and handle design of kettlebells also promote grip strength and wrist stability, important for functional activities and sports performance.

Barbells are commonly used for compound exercises that target large muscle groups and promote strength and muscle hypertrophy.

Squats, deadlifts, bench presses, and overhead presses with barbells allow for progressive overload, where increasing weight challenges muscles to adapt and grow stronger. Barbells also provide stability and support during heavy lifts, making them suitable for strength training programs aimed at developing functional strength and power.

Functional Training Machines and Tools (TRX, Resistance Bands)

Functional training machines and tools add diversity and challenge to functional workouts, offering unique ways to target muscles and movement patterns. TRX suspension trainers, consisting of adjustable straps and handles, utilize body weight and gravity to create resistance in various exercises. TRX rows, chest presses, planks, and mountain climbers engage core stability and functional strength while improving balance and coordination.

Resistance bands, available in different levels of resistance, provide portable and versatile options for functional training. Band exercises such as banded squats, clamshells, lateral walks, and biceps curls target specific muscle groups while also improving flexibility and joint mobility.

The variable resistance of bands allows for progressive overload and accommodates individual fitness levels and goals.

Incorporating functional training machines like cable machines and stability balls adds further variety and challenge to workouts. Cable machines offer adjustable resistance and multiple attachment options for exercises such as cable rows, woodchops, and cable twists, enhancing functional strength and muscular endurance. Stability balls, used for exercises like stability ball squats, planks, and bridges, improve core stability, balance, and proprioception.

Overall, functional fitness equipment provides a diverse and effective means of improving functional strength, mobility, and overall fitness. By incorporating a variety of equipment and exercises into training programs, individuals can enhance their performance in daily activities, sports, and functional movements while reducing the risk of injuries through balanced muscle development and improved movement patterns.

CHAPTER 7
Programming And Periodization

Programming and periodization are fundamental concepts in Functional Fitness that play a crucial role in achieving long-term progress and reaching fitness goals effectively. In this discussion, we'll delve into the principles of Functional Fitness programming, the process of designing workouts tailored to different goals such as strength, endurance, and mobility, and explore various periodization strategies aimed at optimizing performance and avoiding plateaus.

Principles of Functional Fitness Programming

Functional Fitness programming is grounded in several key principles that guide the design and structure of workouts. These principles are essential for ensuring balanced and comprehensive training while minimizing the risk of injury. One fundamental principle is specificity, which emphasizes the importance of tailoring exercises to mimic real-life movements and activities. By focusing on movements that are relevant to daily life or specific sports, Functional Fitness programs can enhance functional strength and performance.

Progressive overload is another critical principle in Functional Fitness programming. It involves gradually increasing the intensity, volume, or complexity of exercises over time to challenge the body and stimulate adaptation.

This principle is central to improving strength, endurance, and mobility as it ensures that the body continues to progress and adapt to new stimuli.

Variation and diversity are also key principles in Functional Fitness programming. Including a variety of exercises, movement patterns, and training modalities helps prevent boredom, stimulates different muscle groups, and reduces the risk of overuse injuries.

Additionally, variation keeps workouts engaging and enjoyable, motivating individuals to stay consistent with their training.

Individualization is another principle that underscores the importance of tailoring workouts to individual needs, goals, and fitness levels.

An effective Functional Fitness program considers factors such as age, fitness background, injury history, and specific goals to create personalized workouts that optimize results and minimize the risk of setbacks.

Finally, recovery and rest are crucial principles in Functional Fitness programming. Adequate rest and recovery periods allow the body to repair and rebuild muscle tissue, prevent burnout, and reduce the risk of overtraining.

Including rest days, incorporating active recovery activities, and prioritizing sleep are integral aspects of a well-rounded Functional Fitness program.

Designing Workouts for Different Goals

One of the strengths of Functional Fitness programming lies in its versatility and ability to cater to a wide range of fitness goals.

Whether the objective is to build strength, improve endurance, enhance mobility, or achieve a combination of these goals, designing effective workouts involves understanding the specific requirements and adaptations associated with each goal.

For strength-focused workouts, emphasis is placed on compound movements that target multiple muscle groups simultaneously. Exercises such as squats, deadlifts, bench presses, and rows are commonly incorporated to develop overall strength and functional capacity.

Additionally, progressive overload principles are applied by gradually increasing resistance, volume, or intensity to continually challenge the muscles and promote strength gains.

Endurance-based workouts in Functional Fitness typically involve cardiovascular exercises aimed at improving aerobic capacity and stamina.

Activities such as running, cycling, rowing, and high-intensity interval training (HIIT) are commonly included to enhance cardiovascular fitness. Structuring workouts with varying intensities, intervals, and recovery periods helps optimize endurance gains while preventing overtraining.

Mobility-focused workouts in Functional Fitness are designed to improve flexibility, joint range of motion, and overall movement quality.

These workouts often incorporate dynamic stretches, mobility drills, and corrective exercises targeting areas of stiffness or limitation. Emphasis is placed on proper form, controlled movements, and gradual progression to enhance mobility without compromising joint stability or risking injury.

Periodization Strategies for Long-Term Progress

Periodization is a systematic approach to structuring workouts over time, typically divided into specific phases or cycles to optimize performance, prevent plateaus, and reduce the risk of overtraining. In Functional Fitness programming, several periodization strategies are commonly used to facilitate long-term progress and adaptation.

Linear periodization is a traditional approach that involves gradually increasing intensity and decreasing volume over time. Workouts are structured in phases, starting with higher volume and lower intensity during the base phase, then progressing to lower volume and higher intensity during the strength and peaking phases.

This approach allows for progressive overload while ensuring adequate recovery and adaptation.

Undulating periodization, also known as nonlinear periodization, involves varying intensity and volume within shorter timeframes, such as weekly or biweekly cycles. This approach provides greater flexibility and variation in workouts, allowing for more frequent changes in stimulus and preventing adaptation plateaus. Undulating periodization is particularly effective for individuals who prefer diverse training stimuli and faster progression.

Block periodization divides training into distinct blocks, each focusing on specific fitness qualities or goals. For example, a strength block may prioritize heavy lifting and maximal strength development, followed by a power block emphasizing explosive movements and speed. This approach allows for concentrated efforts on different aspects of fitness while still incorporating elements of progressive overload and variation.

Concurrent periodization combines multiple fitness qualities within the same training cycle, allowing for the simultaneous development of strength, endurance, and other attributes. This approach is often used in Functional Fitness programs to address the multifaceted nature of fitness and performance requirements.

By strategically balancing different types of workouts within each week or phase, concurrent periodization can lead to comprehensive improvements in overall fitness.

In conclusion, effective Functional Fitness programming involves applying principles such as specificity, progressive overload, variation, individualization, and recovery. Designing workouts tailored to different goals requires understanding the specific demands and adaptations associated with strength, endurance, and mobility training. Implementing periodization strategies such as linear, undulating, block, or concurrent periodization is essential for long-term progress, performance optimization, and preventing training plateaus. By incorporating these principles and strategies, individuals can create well-rounded and sustainable Functional Fitness programs that support their fitness goals and overall health.

CHAPTER 8
Nutrition For Functional Fitness

Functional fitness is not just about the exercises you do; it's also about how you fuel your body to perform optimally. Nutrition plays a crucial role in supporting the demands of functional training, providing the energy, nutrients, and hydration necessary for enhanced performance, recovery, and overall well-being.

Nutritional Requirements for Functional Athletes

Functional athletes have unique nutritional needs compared to traditional athletes due to the diverse movements and intensity levels involved in functional training. Their bodies require a balanced intake of macronutrients (carbohydrates, proteins, and fats) and micronutrients (vitamins and minerals) to support muscle function, energy production, and recovery. Carbohydrates are particularly important as they serve as the primary fuel source during high-intensity workouts, while proteins are essential for muscle repair and growth. Healthy fats play a role in hormone regulation and overall cellular health, contributing to sustained energy levels and performance. Functional athletes should aim for a well-rounded diet that includes a variety of whole foods to meet these nutritional requirements.

Pre-Workout and Post-Workout Nutrition

Optimizing nutrition around workouts is crucial for maximizing performance and recovery.

Pre-workout nutrition focuses on providing the body with the energy and nutrients it needs to sustain intensity and endurance during training sessions. This typically involves consuming a balanced meal or snack containing carbohydrates for immediate energy, proteins for muscle support, and some fats for sustained energy release.

Timing is also essential, with most athletes benefiting from eating 1-2 hours before exercise to allow for digestion and nutrient absorption.

Post-workout nutrition is equally important, as it plays a significant role in recovery and muscle repair. Consuming a combination of carbohydrates and proteins within the post-exercise window (typically within 30 minutes to an hour after training) helps replenish glycogen stores, reduce muscle breakdown, and promote muscle protein synthesis. Fast-digesting carbohydrates like fruits or sports drinks are often recommended alongside lean protein sources such as chicken, fish, or plant-based options like legumes or tofu.

Hydration and Recovery Strategies

Hydration is fundamental for maintaining performance and preventing dehydration, especially during intense functional workouts. Fluid needs vary depending on factors such as exercise intensity, duration, and environmental conditions. Functional athletes should prioritize staying hydrated throughout the day and during training sessions by drinking water regularly. Electrolytes, such as sodium, potassium, and magnesium, are also crucial for maintaining fluid balance and muscle function, particularly in prolonged or high-sweat activities. Sports drinks or electrolyte supplements can be beneficial during extended workouts or in hot environments to replace lost electrolytes.

Recovery strategies extend beyond nutrition and hydration to include aspects like rest, sleep, and active recovery techniques. Adequate rest and sleep are essential for muscle repair and growth, hormone regulation, and overall recovery from training stress. Incorporating active recovery activities such as light stretching, foam rolling, or low-intensity exercise can enhance blood flow, reduce muscle soreness, and improve recovery between workouts. Balancing training intensity with proper nutrition, hydration, and recovery strategies is key to optimizing performance and long-term progress in functional fitness.

CHAPTER 9
Injury Prevention And Recovery

Common Injuries in Functional Fitness

Functional fitness training is highly beneficial for improving overall strength, flexibility, and mobility. However, like any physical activity, it also carries a risk of injuries, particularly if proper precautions are not taken. Understanding the common injuries that can occur in functional fitness is crucial for designing effective injury prevention strategies and promoting safe training practices.

One of the most prevalent injuries in functional fitness is muscle strain or sprain. These injuries often occur due to overexertion, improper form during exercises, or inadequate warm-up. Commonly affected areas include the back, shoulders, knees, and ankles. Symptoms may include pain, swelling, and limited range of motion. To prevent muscle strains, athletes should focus on proper technique, gradually increase intensity and load, and incorporate adequate rest and recovery into their training routines.

Another frequent injury is joint-related, such as tendonitis or bursitis. These conditions result from repetitive movements, overuse, or poor biomechanics. For example, shoulder tendonitis can develop from excessive overhead pressing without proper shoulder stability and mobility. Prevention strategies involve incorporating variety into workouts, performing joint-specific mobility drills, and addressing muscle imbalances through targeted exercises.

In addition to muscle and joint injuries, functional fitness enthusiasts may also experience lower back pain. This can stem from poor posture, weak core muscles, or improper lifting techniques.

Core stability exercises, correct lifting mechanics, and maintaining a neutral spine during exercises are essential for preventing lower back issues.

Moreover, addressing mobility limitations in the hips and thoracic spine can alleviate stress on the lower back.

Prehabilitation Exercises

Prehabilitation, or prehab, refers to proactive measures taken to prevent injuries before they occur. Incorporating prehabilitation exercises into a functional fitness program is essential for enhancing joint stability, improving movement patterns, and reducing the risk of injuries.

These exercises focus on strengthening muscles, enhancing flexibility, and promoting proper biomechanics.

For shoulder prehabilitation, exercises targeting the rotator cuff muscles are vital. External and internal rotation exercises using resistance bands or light weights help strengthen the rotator cuff and stabilize the shoulder joint. Scapular stabilization drills, such as prone Ys and Ts, improve shoulder blade control and function, reducing the likelihood of shoulder injuries during pressing and pulling movements.

To prevent knee injuries, prehabilitation exercises should address quadriceps, hamstrings, and hip muscles. Squats, lunges, and leg press variations strengthen the lower body while promoting proper knee alignment. Additionally, hip abduction and adduction exercises improve hip stability, reducing stress on the knees during lateral movements and pivoting actions.

For lower back prehabilitation, core strengthening exercises are paramount. Planks, bird dogs, and dead bug variations target the deep core muscles, enhancing spinal stability and reducing the risk of lower back pain. Incorporating exercises that promote hip mobility and thoracic spine extension also contributes to a healthier spine and improved functional movement patterns.

Recovery Techniques (Foam Rolling, Stretching, Sleep)

Effective recovery is essential for optimizing performance, reducing muscle soreness, and preventing injuries in functional fitness. Incorporating various recovery techniques into post-workout routines promotes muscle relaxation, enhances flexibility, and facilitates tissue repair and regeneration.

Foam rolling, also known as self-myofascial release, is a popular recovery technique used to release muscle tightness and improve tissue mobility.

By applying pressure to specific areas using a foam roller or massage ball, athletes can target trigger points and knots, promoting blood flow and reducing muscle tension. Foam rolling sessions targeting major muscle groups such as the quadriceps, hamstrings, calves, and back can aid in post-exercise recovery.

Stretching is another valuable component of recovery that helps maintain or improve flexibility and joint range of motion. Dynamic stretching before workouts prepares muscles for activity by increasing blood flow and activating the neuromuscular system. Static stretching after workouts or on rest days helps elongate muscles, improve muscle relaxation, and prevent stiffness. Incorporating a combination of dynamic and static stretches targeting major muscle groups ensures comprehensive flexibility maintenance.

Quality sleep is often overlooked but plays a critical role in recovery and overall well-being. During sleep, the body undergoes essential processes such as hormone regulation, tissue repair, and memory consolidation.

Adequate sleep duration (7-9 hours for most adults) and quality (uninterrupted, restorative sleep cycles) are crucial for optimal physical and mental recovery. Establishing a consistent sleep schedule, creating a relaxing bedtime routine, and optimizing the sleep environment (e.g., dark, quiet, comfortable) contribute to improved recovery outcomes.

understanding common injuries, incorporating prehabilitation exercises, and utilizing effective recovery techniques are integral aspects of injury prevention and promoting long-term success in functional fitness training.

By prioritizing proper technique, progressive training, and comprehensive recovery strategies, individuals can enjoy the benefits of functional fitness while minimizing the risk of injuries.

CHAPTER 10
Monitoring Progress And Goal Setting

Tracking progress and setting goals are crucial aspects of any fitness program, including Functional Fitness. These practices not only provide a clear roadmap for improvement but also help individuals stay motivated and accountable.

In Functional Fitness, monitoring progress goes beyond just looking at physical changes; it involves assessing functional movement, strength gains, mobility improvements, and overall performance enhancements. This comprehensive approach ensures that individuals not only look fit but also function optimally in their daily activities and sports.

One of the key methods for tracking progress in Functional Fitness is through functional movement assessments. These assessments evaluate how well an individual can perform fundamental movements such as squats, hinges, pushes, pulls, and rotations.

By regularly assessing these movements, trainers and practitioners can identify areas of strength and weakness, track improvements over time, and tailor training programs to address specific needs.

Functional movement assessments are often part of a comprehensive evaluation process that includes mobility tests, flexibility assessments, and performance metrics related to cardiovascular fitness and muscular endurance.

In addition to movement assessments, objective measures such as strength testing, mobility measurements, and endurance assessments are vital for monitoring progress in Functional Fitness.

Strength tests like one-rep max (1RM) for key lifts such as squats, deadlifts, and presses provide quantitative data on muscular strength gains. Mobility measurements, such as joint range of motion assessments and flexibility tests, track improvements in mobility and flexibility. Endurance assessments, including timed workouts or distance challenges, gauge cardiovascular fitness progress.

These objective measures, when combined with subjective feedback from clients regarding how they feel during workouts and in daily life, paint a comprehensive picture of progress in Functional Fitness.

Setting SMART goals is another essential component of effective progress tracking and goal setting in Functional Fitness. SMART goals are Specific, Measurable, Achievable, Relevant, and Time-bound.

Specific goals outline precisely what the individual wants to achieve, such as increasing squat depth or improving shoulder mobility.

Measurable goals provide a quantifiable metric to track progress, such as adding 10 pounds to a lift or increasing flexibility by a certain degree.

Achievable goals are realistic and attainable within a given timeframe, considering the individual's current fitness level and capabilities.

Relevant goals align with the individual's overall fitness objectives and Functional Fitness priorities. Time-bound goals have a defined timeline for achievement, which creates a sense of urgency and accountability.

When setting SMART goals in Functional Fitness, it's essential to consider both short-term and long-term objectives. Short-term goals focus on immediate improvements, such as increasing weight lifted or improving form in a specific exercise.

Long-term goals encompass broader fitness outcomes, such as enhancing overall functional movement patterns, achieving specific performance milestones, or participating in targeted sports or activities. By breaking down long-term goals into manageable short-term objectives, individuals can maintain motivation and track progress effectively.

Adjusting training plans based on progress is a dynamic process in Functional Fitness.

As individuals make progress toward their goals, it's essential to reassess and adapt training programs to ensure continued growth and prevent plateaus. This adaptation may involve increasing training intensity, adjusting exercise volume and frequency, incorporating new exercises or variations, modifying recovery strategies, or addressing any emerging limitations or imbalances.

Periodic reassessments of functional movement, strength, mobility, and endurance help determine the effectiveness of current training protocols and identify areas for modification.

For example, if an individual has significantly improved lower body strength but struggles with upper body mobility, the training plan may be adjusted to prioritize mobility drills and corrective exercises for the upper body.

Likewise, if cardiovascular endurance has plateaued, introducing interval training or increasing workout intensity can stimulate further adaptations.

Moreover, feedback from clients regarding their experience, preferences, and challenges during training sessions is invaluable in refining training plans. Communication between trainers, practitioners, and clients fosters a collaborative approach to goal setting and program adjustments, ensuring that training remains aligned with individual needs and objectives.

Monitoring progress and setting SMART goals are integral components of effective Functional Fitness programming. By tracking functional movement, strength gains, mobility improvements, and endurance enhancements, individuals can assess their progress comprehensively.

Setting SMART goals provides a structured framework for goal setting that is specific, measurable, achievable, relevant, and time-bound. Adjusting training plans based on progress involves dynamic adaptations to ensure continued growth, prevent plateaus, and address evolving fitness needs. This iterative process of progress tracking, goal setting, and program adjustment supports ongoing improvement and success in Functional Fitness endeavors.

CHAPTER 11
Advanced Functional Training Techniques

Advanced Functional Training Techniques encompass a range of specialized exercises and methodologies designed to enhance athletic performance, improve functional movement patterns, and target specific aspects of physical fitness such as power, agility, speed, and sport-specific skills.

These techniques go beyond basic exercises and require a deeper understanding of biomechanics, neuromuscular coordination, and training principles to achieve optimal results. In this section, we will delve into Plyometric Training for Power, Agility, Speed Drills, and Sport-Specific Functional Training, exploring their benefits, methodologies, and applications in athletic development.

Plyometric Training for Power

Plyometric training is a dynamic form of exercise that focuses on rapid muscle contractions to improve explosive power, speed, and overall athletic performance. It involves quick, powerful movements that utilize the stretch-shortening cycle of muscles, enhancing their ability to generate force rapidly. The key principle behind plyometrics is the utilization of eccentric (lengthening) and concentric (shortening) muscle actions in rapid succession, leading to enhanced neuromuscular coordination and muscular power output.

One of the fundamental concepts in plyometric training is the stretch-shortening cycle, which involves three phases: eccentric (loading), amortization (transition), and concentric (explosive contraction). During the eccentric phase, the muscle lengthens under tension, storing elastic energy. This energy is then released rapidly during the concentric phase, resulting in a powerful contraction. The amortization phase is crucial as it represents the transition between eccentric and concentric actions, where the muscle switches from loading to exploding.

Common plyometric exercises include depth jumps, box jumps, bounding, and medicine ball throws. These exercises are typically performed with maximal effort and minimal ground contact time to maximize power output. Plyometric training is beneficial for athletes involved in sports requiring explosive movements such as basketball, sprinting, volleyball, and martial arts.

Agility and Speed Drills

Agility and speed are essential components of athletic performance, especially in sports that demand quick changes in direction, acceleration, and deceleration. Agility drills focus on improving multi-directional movements, reactive ability, and footwork, enhancing an athlete's ability to change direction swiftly and efficiently. Speed drills, on the other hand, target linear speed, acceleration, and sprinting mechanics to increase overall speed and velocity.

Agility drills often incorporate cone drills, ladder drills, shuttle runs, and reactive agility drills that simulate game-like scenarios requiring rapid changes in movement patterns. These drills challenge proprioception, spatial awareness, and coordination, improving an athlete's ability to navigate complex environments and respond quickly to stimuli.

Speed drills encompass techniques such as sprint intervals, resisted sprinting (using sleds or resistance bands), and technique-focused drills to optimize running mechanics. Proper sprinting form, including arm drive, knee lift, and body lean, is emphasized to maximize speed and efficiency.

Both agility and speed drills play a crucial role in enhancing athletic performance by improving reaction time, agility, acceleration, deceleration, and overall speed capabilities. They are particularly beneficial for sports such as soccer, football, tennis, and rugby, where quick changes in direction and explosive bursts of speed are essential for success.

Sport-Specific Functional Training

Sport-specific functional training is tailored to the specific movement patterns, biomechanics, and demands of a particular sport. It involves exercises and drills that mimic the actions and skills required during competition, targeting muscles and movement patterns relevant to the sport's performance requirements.

This type of training aims to improve sport-specific skills, muscular strength, endurance, and overall athletic ability within the context of the athlete's chosen sport.

For example, a basketball player may engage in sport-specific functional training that includes dribbling drills, shooting techniques, agility exercises for quick lateral movements, and strength training focusing on lower body explosiveness and core stability. Similarly, a soccer player's training regimen may include ball control drills, sprint intervals, agility ladder work, and lower body strength exercises to improve kicking power and agility on the field.

Sport-specific functional training is highly individualized and takes into account the unique physical demands and movement patterns of each sport. It often involves a combination of strength training, plyometric, agility drills, flexibility work, and sport-specific skills training to optimize athletic performance and reduce the risk of injury.

By incorporating sport-specific functional training into their regimen, athletes can improve their overall performance, enhance skill proficiency, and develop the physical attributes necessary for success in their chosen sport. This type of training not only enhances athletic ability but also promotes functional movement patterns that translate directly to improved performance during competitive situations.

Advanced Functional Training Techniques such as Plyometric Training for Power, Agility, Speed

Drills, and Sport-Specific Functional Training are integral components of athletic development and performance enhancement. These techniques target specific aspects of physical fitness, including explosive power, agility, speed, and sport-specific skills, allowing athletes to optimize their performance and excel in competitive environments. Integrating these advanced training methodologies into a comprehensive training program can lead to significant improvements in athletic ability, functional movement patterns, and overall success in sports and athletic endeavors.

CHAPTER 12
Mental Conditioning And Mindfulness

Mental conditioning and mindfulness play crucial roles in achieving peak performance and sustained progress in Functional Fitness. This section delves into the concepts of mental strength, mindfulness practices, and strategies for overcoming common hurdles like plateaus and mental blocks.

Mental Strength in Functional Fitness

Mental strength in Functional Fitness encompasses a range of psychological attributes that contribute to resilience, focus, and determination during workouts and training programs. It involves the ability to stay motivated, manage stress effectively, and maintain a positive mindset despite challenges. Mental strength is cultivated through consistent practice, self-awareness, and strategies such as goal setting, visualization, and positive self-talk.

One key aspect of mental strength is resilience, which refers to the capacity to bounce back from setbacks and adapt to changing circumstances.

In Functional Fitness, where progress often involves facing physical and mental barriers, resilience becomes a fundamental quality.

It enables athletes to persevere through tough workouts, recover from injuries, and stay committed to long-term goals despite obstacles.

Another component of mental strength is focus and concentration. In Functional Fitness routines, especially during complex movements or high-intensity intervals, the ability to maintain focus is critical for safety and optimal performance. Techniques like mindfulness meditation, breath control, and visualization exercises can enhance focus and reduce distractions during workouts.

Moreover, mental strength involves emotional regulation and stress management.

Intense workouts and competitive environments can trigger stress and anxiety, impacting performance and recovery.

Developing coping strategies such as deep breathing, progressive muscle relaxation, and cognitive reframing can help athletes manage stress effectively and maintain emotional balance during training sessions.

Mindfulness Practices for Performance Enhancement

Mindfulness practices are valuable tools for improving performance, enhancing self-awareness, and promoting overall well-being in Functional Fitness. Mindfulness involves being fully present in the moment, without judgment or distraction, and can be cultivated through various techniques such as meditation, body scan exercises, and mindful movement.

One of the primary benefits of mindfulness in Functional Fitness is improved body awareness. By paying attention to bodily sensations, movement patterns, and posture, athletes can identify areas of strength and weakness, prevent injuries, and refine their technique for optimal performance. Mindful movement practices, such as yoga and tai chi, can also enhance flexibility, mobility, and coordination, complementing Functional Fitness training.

Furthermore, mindfulness helps athletes develop a non-reactive mindset, enabling them to respond calmly and effectively to challenges during workouts.

By cultivating acceptance and resilience, athletes can navigate setbacks, injuries, and plateaus with greater ease and perseverance. Mindfulness also fosters mental clarity and decision-making skills, enhancing performance in complex movements and strategic training plans.

Incorporating mindfulness into daily routines, such as pre-workout rituals or cooldown sessions, can enhance the overall quality of training and promote recovery.

Techniques like mindful breathing, body-awareness exercises, and visualization can be integrated into warm-ups, cooldowns, and recovery sessions to promote relaxation, focus, and mental resilience.

Overcoming Plateaus and Mental Blocks

Plateaus and mental blocks are common challenges encountered in Functional Fitness, where progress can stagnate despite consistent effort and training. Overcoming these obstacles requires a combination of mental strategies, adaptive training approaches, and goal-oriented planning.

One approach to overcoming plateaus is periodization, which involves varying training intensity, volume, and exercises over time to stimulate adaptation and prevent stagnation.

By incorporating progressive overload principles, deload phases, and strategic rest periods, athletes can break through plateaus and continue making gains in strength, endurance, and performance.

Additionally, addressing mental blocks involves identifying underlying beliefs, fears, or negative thought patterns that may be limiting progress. Cognitive-behavioral techniques, such as cognitive restructuring and self-efficacy building, can help athletes challenge and reframe unproductive thoughts, boost confidence, and foster a growth mindset toward training and performance goals.

Moreover, seeking feedback, support, and guidance from coaches, peers, or mental health professionals can provide valuable insights and strategies for overcoming plateaus and mental blocks. Collaborative goal-setting, performance evaluations, and tailored training programs can help athletes navigate challenges, stay motivated, and sustain long-term progress in Functional Fitness.

Mental conditioning and mindfulness practices are integral components of success in Functional Fitness, contributing to mental strength, performance enhancement, and resilience in the face of obstacles.

By cultivating a positive mindset, developing self-awareness, and utilizing effective strategies, athletes can optimize their training experience, achieve peak performance, and overcome challenges to reach their full potential in Functional Fitness.

CHAPTER 13
Special Populations And Functional Fitness

Functional fitness is a dynamic approach to exercise that emphasizes movements and activities that mimic real-life functions and improve overall functional abilities. When applied to special populations, such as older adults, individuals undergoing rehabilitation, pregnant women, or those with disabilities, functional fitness takes on a tailored and nuanced form to address specific needs while promoting health and well-being.

Functional fitness for older adults is a crucial aspect of promoting healthy aging and maintaining independence. As individuals age, there is a natural decline in muscle mass, strength, flexibility, and balance, which can increase the risk of falls and injuries. Functional fitness programs for older adults focus on exercises that improve strength, balance, flexibility, and coordination, all essential components for maintaining daily activities and quality of life.

These programs often incorporate bodyweight exercises, resistance training with light weights or bands, balance exercises, and flexibility drills.

The goal is to enhance functional capacity, promote joint health, and reduce the risk of age-related mobility issues.

Rehabilitation is another area where functional fitness plays a vital role in restoring movement, strength, and function after injury or surgery. Functional rehabilitation training involves a personalized approach that addresses specific limitations and goals.

Physical therapists and rehabilitation specialists design programs that target the affected area(s) while also considering the individual's overall functional needs. This may include exercises to improve range of motion, strengthen muscles, enhance proprioception, and facilitate proper movement patterns.

By focusing on functional movements relevant to daily activities, rehabilitation programs aim to optimize recovery and restore functional independence.

Tailoring workouts for specific needs, such as pregnancy or disabilities, requires a thoughtful and individualized approach to ensure safety and effectiveness.

Pregnant women can benefit from modified exercises that support pelvic floor health, maintain core stability, and improve overall strength and flexibility. These workouts typically avoid high-impact activities and incorporate prenatal considerations to accommodate changing body mechanics and hormone levels.

Additionally, exercises that promote relaxation and reduce stress can be beneficial during pregnancy.

For individuals with disabilities, functional fitness programs aim to improve functional capacity, mobility, and quality of life.

This may involve adaptive exercises, assistive devices, and specialized techniques to address unique challenges and limitations. The focus is on enhancing independence, promoting social inclusion, and empowering individuals to engage in physical activity that suits their abilities and goals.

Functional fitness for special populations highlights the importance of personalized and targeted exercise programs to address specific needs, promote health, and enhance overall well-being.

Whether it's older adults, individuals in rehabilitation, pregnant women, or those with disabilities, functional fitness offers a holistic approach that fosters functional capacity, movement quality, and a higher quality of life.

Conclusion

The book on Functional Fitness covers a wide range of topics essential for understanding and implementing functional training.

It delves into the definition and benefits of Functional Fitness, explores various functional movement patterns like squatting, hinging, pushing, pulling, rotational exercises, and anti-rotational exercises.

Core stability and strength are emphasized with detailed exercises and progressions. Mobility and flexibility training are discussed, highlighting the importance of joint mobility and dynamic warm-ups.

Cardiovascular training, including HIIT and endurance workouts, is integrated into functional fitness routines. The manual also explores functional fitness equipment such as bodyweight exercises, dumbbells, kettlebells, and machines like TRX and resistance bands.

Programming and periodization principles are outlined for designing effective workouts based on different goals.

Nutrition guidelines for functional athletes, injury prevention strategies, monitoring progress, goal setting techniques, and advanced training methods like plyometric and agility drills are covered. Mental conditioning and mindfulness practices for performance enhancement, as well as considerations for special populations like older adults and individuals undergoing rehabilitation, are also discussed.

www.ingramcontent.com/pod-product-compliance
Lightning Source LLC
Chambersburg PA
CBHW050119230526
45470CB00004B/1897